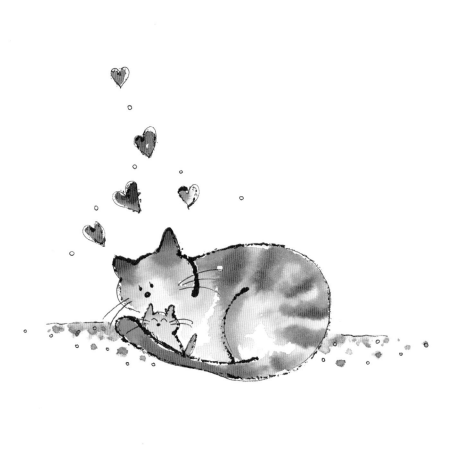

From the first *smile*,

to the first steps, the first words...

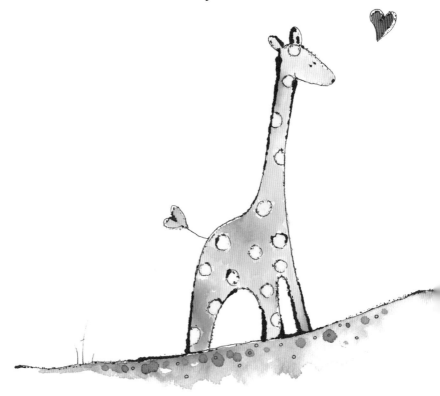

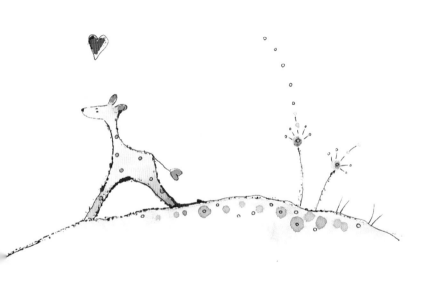

each moment is cherished FOREVER.

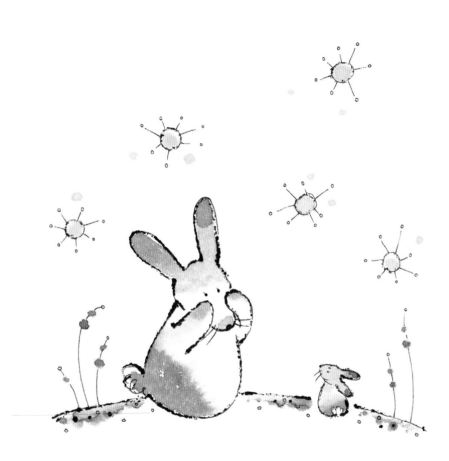

You'll say '*peepo*!' a thousand times –

make up silly songs or DANCE around the room –

if it makes your baby smile!

To cradle a baby close, and watch them sleep,

so *perfect*, so precious...

nothing is more peaceful or more LOVELY!

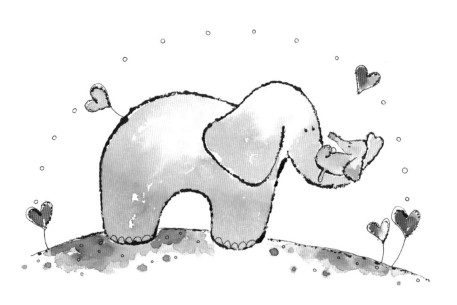

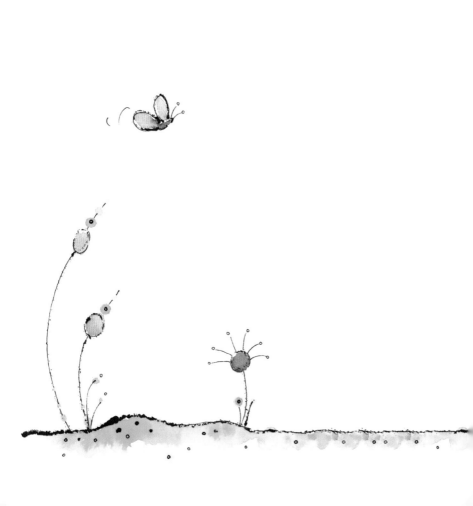

Your baby is here at last,

and SUDDENLY nothing is as it was –

a new life, a new *family* begins.

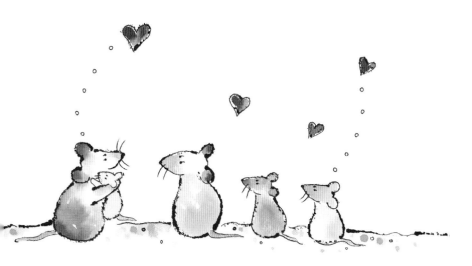

KISSES on cheeks and baby coos,

kisses on hands and baby smiles,

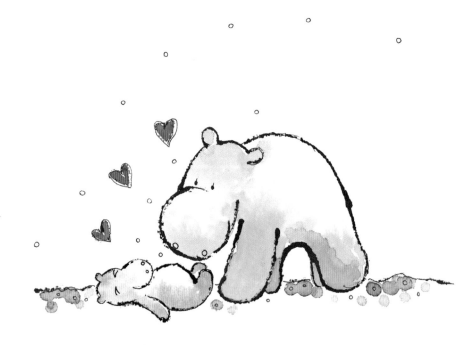

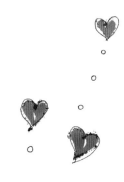

kisses on tummy and baby *giggles* –

over and over, again and again!

How can it be?

A tiny baby is so *adorable*, so sweet...

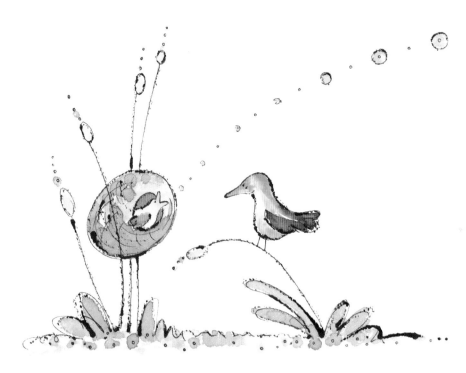

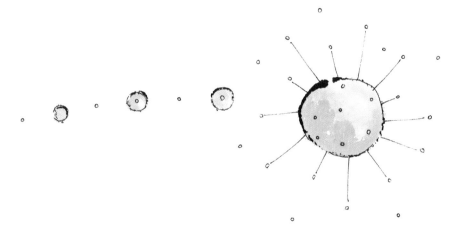

yet sometimes so impossibly LOUD!

Your *little* baby,

safe in your arms,

is the most precious thing in the WORLD!

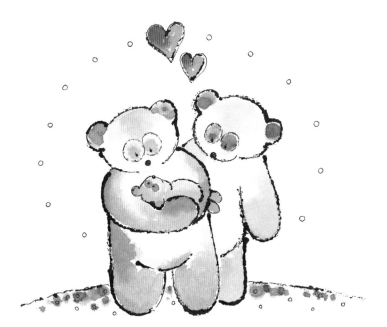

When your baby smiles,

suddenly ALL troubles are forgotten –

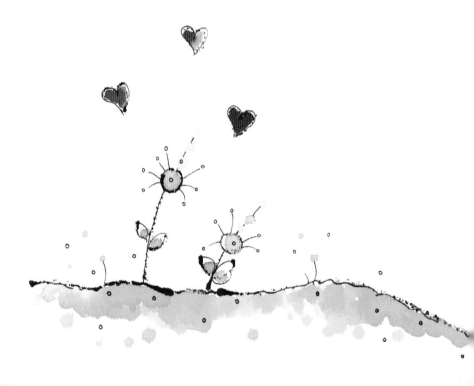

everything is calm,

and just as it should be!

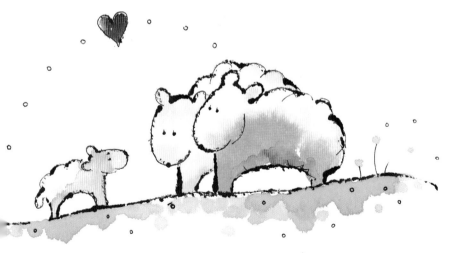

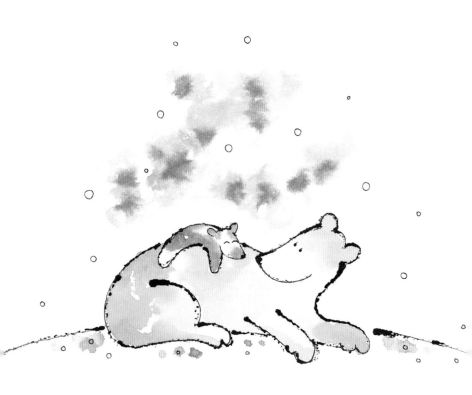

Happiness is...

a moment's rest, a cup of tea

and your baby sleeping *peacefully*!

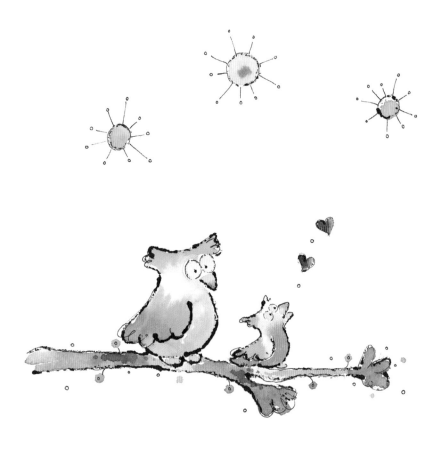

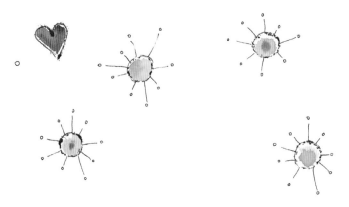

EACH new thing your baby does

makes you so *proud*!

A *baby* takes so much –

of your time, your energy, your patience!

And yet, in return, gives so much JOY.

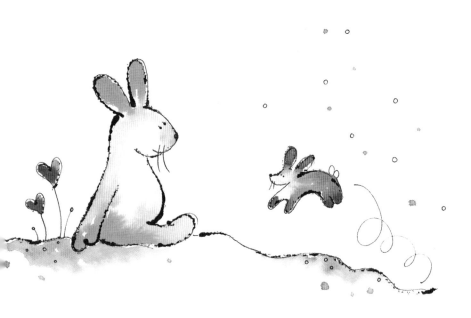

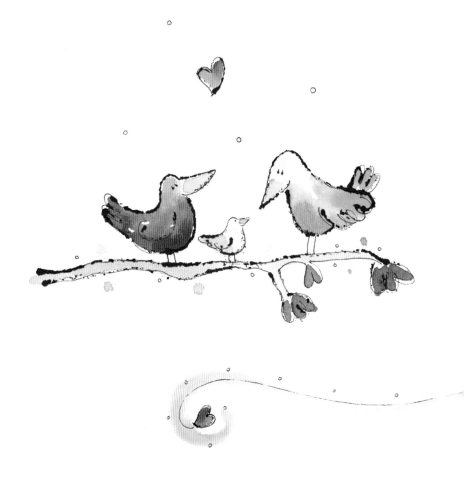

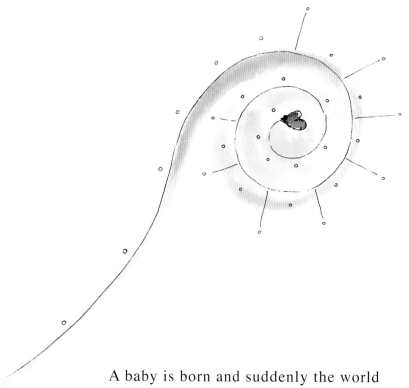

A baby is born and suddenly the world

seems FULL of new hope,

new dreams and *endless* possibilities.

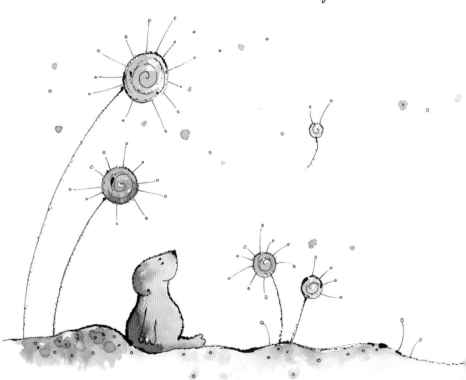

and a **PERFECT**, tiny button nose!

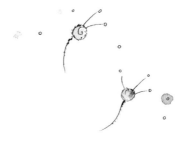

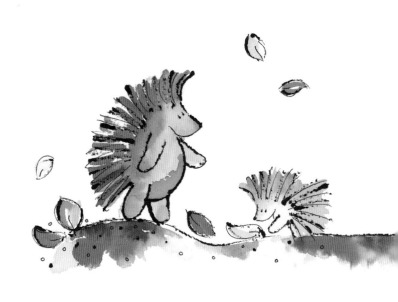

Every baby is a miracle –

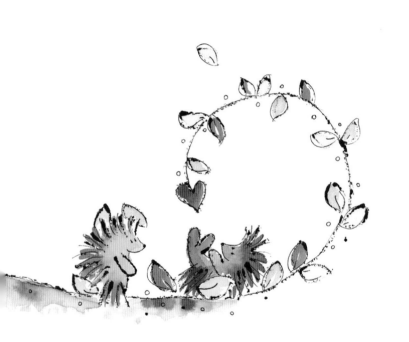

utterly unique and AMAZING!

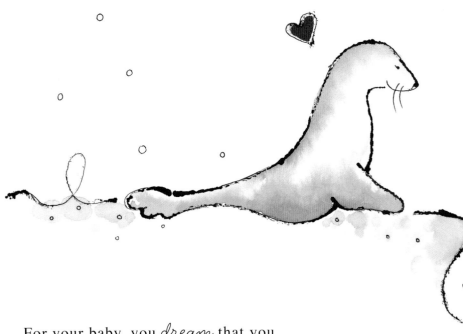

For your baby, you *dream* that you

will ALWAYS be there to give comfort and advice,

and to cheer them on to follow their *dreams*!

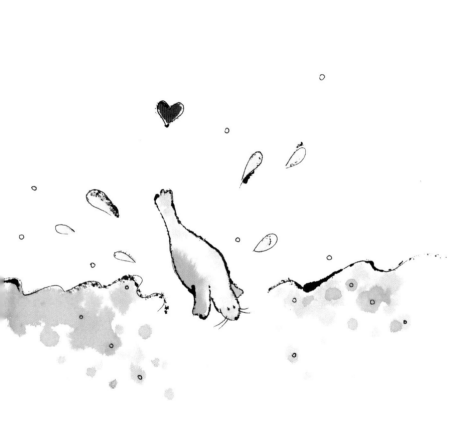

A day with your baby may be *messy* and chaotic...

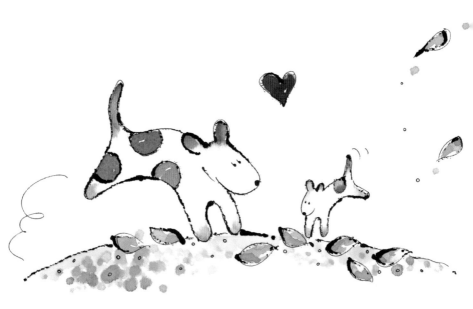

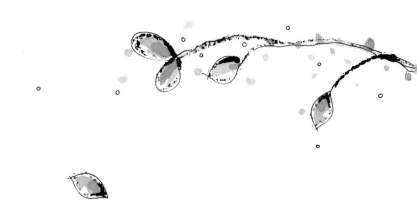

but it's always full of lovely SILLINESS!

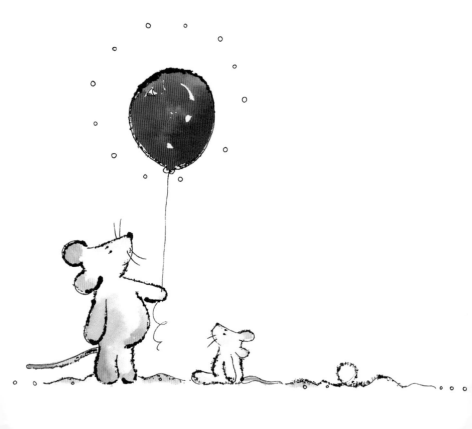

To a baby, EVERYTHING in the world

is new and so *exciting*!

Babies bring *many* things,

but above all else, they bring LOVE!

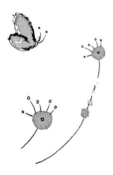

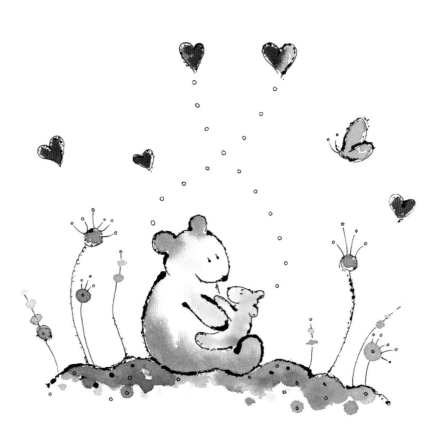